DUKAN DIET ESSENTIALS

Unlock the Secrets of Four Phases, Transform Your Relationship with Food, and Embrace a Healthier, Happier You

ALSO ADDED
2 BONUS (A FREE COOKBOOK)

Sara Barrett

Copyright

© 2023 by Sara Berrett

This book is a work of fiction. Names, characters, places, and incidents are the product of the author's imagination or are used fictitiously. Any resemblance to actual events, locales, or persons, living or dead, is coincidental.

About Author

Sara Barrett is a passionate advocate for holistic well-being, with a keen focus on nutrition, fitness, and the unique needs of endomorphs. As a certified nutritionist and fitness enthusiast, Sara brings a wealth of knowledge and personal experience to her writing.

With a background in nutritional sciences and a dedication to promoting a balanced and joyful approach to healthy living, Jane has empowered individuals on their journeys to wellness. Her philosophy revolves around embracing individuality, finding joy in nourishing the body, and fostering a positive relationship with food and exercise.

Beyond her credentials, Sara's love for creating delicious, nutritious recipes is contagious. Through her writing, she invites readers to explore a world where every meal is a celebration and every workout is an opportunity to move with purpose.

"Dukan Diet Essentials" is the culmination of Sara's expertise, personal journey, and commitment to empowering individuals to thrive in their unique bodies. Her warm and relatable approach makes this book not just a guide to nutrition and fitness but a companion on the path to a healthier, happier life.

TABLE OF CONTENT

INTRODUCTION

Unveiling the Dukan Diet

In a world brimming with an array of diet trends promising quick fixes and miraculous transformations, the Dukan Diet stands as a beacon of science-backed efficacy. Conceived by the visionary French nutritionist, Dr. Pierre Dukan, this revolutionary approach to weight loss transcends fads, offering a structured yet flexible path toward achieving lasting results.

As we embark on this journey through the Dukan Diet, it's essential to grasp the fundamental philosophy that sets it apart. Dr. Dukan's creation is not just a diet; it's a transformative lifestyle that empowers individuals to take control of their weight, health, and well-being.

The Visionary behind the Diet

Dr. Pierre Dukan, with decades of expertise in nutrition, crafted this methodology with a deep understanding of the complexities of weight management. His vision was to create a sustainable system that not only sheds excess pounds but also instills a sense of discipline and balance in one's relationship with food.

A Glimpse into Success

Before we delve into the intricacies of each phase, let's take a moment to witness the incredible stories of individuals who, like you, once stood at the threshold of change. Through the Dukan Diet, they not only achieved their weight loss goals but also discovered a newfound vitality and confidence. These success stories are not just testimonials; they are living proof that the Dukan Diet is a transformative journey worth embarking upon.

What Sets the Dukan Diet Apart?

Unlike fleeting diet trends, the Dukan Diet is grounded in four distinct phases —Attack, Cruise, Consolidation, and Stabilization— each meticulously designed to fulfill a specific purpose in your weight loss journey. As we unfold the layers of each phase, you'll discover the logic, science, and methodology behind the Dukan Diet's unparalleled success.

Embarking on Your Dukan Journey

The pages that follow are your guide to understanding, embracing, and successfully navigating the Dukan Diet. From the initial high-impact Attack Phase to the lifelong habits cultivated in the Stabilization Phase, every chapter is a step toward a healthier, more vibrant you.

Are you ready to unlock the secrets to sustainable weight loss and a revitalized lifestyle? Let the Dukan Diet be your compass on this transformative journey—one that promises not just a slimmer figure but a renewed sense of well-being and self-mastery. Welcome to a world where your health takes center stage, and lasting change becomes your reality.

CHAPTER 1

Introduction to Dr. Pierre Dukan and the philosophy behind the Dukan Diet.

In this pivotal chapter, we embark on a fascinating exploration of the esteemed Dr. Pierre Dukan, the visionary founder of the Dukan Diet. Dr. Dukan's remarkable contributions to the field of nutrition and his innovative approach to sustainable weight management have left an indelible mark on the world of dietary science.

We begin by delving into Dr. Pierre Dukan's background, tracing the early influences and experiences that shaped his journey towards becoming a renowned figure in the realm of nutrition and weight loss. From his formative years to his professional education and beyond, we uncover the pivotal milestones that led to the development of the Dukan Diet.

As we peel back the layers of Dr. Dukan's career, we gain insight into his medical expertise, academic achievements, and the profound impact of his research in the field of dietetics. We explore the scientific rigor and clinical foundation that underpins the Dukan Diet, illuminating the evidence-based principles that distinguish it as a leading dietary strategy.

Moreover, we delve into the pivotal moments and epiphanies that sparked Dr. Dukan's visionary creation of the diet, shedding light on the motivations, challenges, and triumphs that accompanied the inception of this groundbreaking approach to weight management.

In this chapter, we also spotlight the research and clinical studies that have validated the efficacy and safety of the Dukan Diet, reinforcing the credibility and scientific rigor that underlie Dr. Dukan's revolutionary dietary methodology.

By the conclusion of this chapter, readers will not only gain a profound understanding of Dr. Pierre Dukan's pioneering contributions to the field of nutrition but will also be inspired by the vision, dedication, and expertise that have propelled the Dukan Diet to the forefront of sustainable weight management strategies.

A glimpse into the success stories that have inspired many to embark on this transformative journey

The Dukan Diet has been a catalyst for remarkable transformations, empowering individuals to achieve astounding weight loss and revitalized well-being. These inspiring narratives serve as beacons of hope, illustrating the profound impact of the Dukan Diet on the lives of those who have embraced its principles with dedication and determination.

From triumphant weight loss achievements to the restoration of confidence and vitality, the success stories of individuals such as Ilene R., Annie F., Courtney K., Sam, Lori V., and many others exemplify the life-altering effects of committing to the Dukan Diet. Their testimonials resonate with authenticity, offering a glimpse into the profound changes experienced through this groundbreaking approach to healthy living.

For instance, Annie F. eloquently articulates her awe-inspiring 125-pound weight loss, capturing the essence of newfound possibilities and personal empowerment. Similarly, the journey of Courtney K. illuminates the transformative realization of regaining control over one's life through the pursuit of wellness and resilience.

These accounts of triumph go beyond mere numbers on a scale, encapsulating the essence of renewed vitality, enhanced self-esteem, and an unwavering commitment to sustainable well-being. The narratives of individuals like Sam, Lori V., and Joanna D. reflect the multifaceted impact of the Dukan Diet, encompassing physical, emotional, and holistic transformation.

Furthermore, the profound testimonials of Matthew K., Hannah, and Jessica W. offer a poignant portrayal of the metamorphosis that arises from embracing the Dukan Diet as a catalyst for positive change. Their journeys stand as testament to the resilience, perseverance, and gratifying rewards that accompany the pursuit of holistic health and well-being.

These narratives serve as a testament to the life-changing potential of the Dukan Diet, igniting a beacon of hope for individuals seeking a sustainable path to weight loss, revitalized health, and renewed vitality. Through these extraordinary testimonials, readers are offered a glimpse into the profound impact of the Dukan Diet, inspiring them to embark on their own transformative journey towards a healthier, more vibrant lifestyle.

Certainly! The success stories shared showcased the transformative impact of the Dukan Diet on individuals who have embraced its principles. These testimonials offer a glimpse into the diverse experiences and remarkable achievements of those who have embarked on their weight loss journeys with the support of the Dukan Diet.

From Jennifer D.'s astounding 135-pound weight loss to Annie F.'s remarkable 125-pound transformation, these success stories underscore the profound impact of the Dukan Diet on individuals' lives. The testimonials also convey the emotional and psychological shifts that accompany significant weight loss, with individuals expressing newfound confidence, vitality, and a renewed sense of self.

Moreover, the testimonials reflect the diverse paths that led individuals to the Dukan Diet, from Ilene R.'s discovery of the diet through a friend's recommendation to Sam's profound commitment to transformation for the sake of his family. These narratives resonate with authenticity and serve as a source of inspiration for readers considering their own wellness journeys

Additionally, the testimonials offer insights into the sustainability and long-term impact of the Dukan Diet, with Lori V.'s experience of being taken off blood pressure and cholesterol medication after six months on the plan, highlighting the holistic health benefits that extend beyond mere weight loss.

The success stories also underscore the diverse approaches and personalized experiences of individuals following the Dukan Diet, from Matthew K.'s dedication to hitting the gym regularly to Hannah's expression of increased energy and vitality.

Overall, the testimonials provide a multifaceted portrayal of the transformative power of the Dukan Diet, offering readers a sense of hope, inspiration, and a testament to the potential for meaningful change through the adoption of a sustainable and personalized approach to wellness.

Teaser of the benefits readers can expect to discover in the upcoming chapters

In the forthcoming chapters of this compelling journey through the world of the Dukan Diet, readers can anticipate an array of enlightening and empowering insights that will revolutionize their approach to weight management and overall well-being.

From unravelling the intricacies of the Dukan Diet's unique four-phase approach to shedding light on the science-backed principles that underpin its effectiveness, readers will gain a comprehensive understanding of how this transformative dietary strategy can catalyze sustainable weight loss and holistic vitality.

Moreover, the upcoming chapters will delve into the nuances of the Dukan Diet's renowned emphasis on lean protein, unveiling the profound impact of this dietary cornerstone on metabolic efficiency, satiety, and muscle preservation. Readers will uncover the compelling science behind the diet's protein-centric philosophy and its potential to redefine their relationship with food and fuel their journey towards a healthier, more vibrant lifestyle.

Furthermore, the chapters will unveil the practical strategies and personalized approaches that empower individuals to navigate the challenges and triumphs of the

Dukan Diet with confidence and resilience. From meal planning and recipe inspiration to navigating social occasions and sustaining long-term success, readers will discover invaluable guidance and resources to fortify their commitment to sustainable well-being.

Additionally, the upcoming chapters will illuminate the profound impact of the Dukan Diet on diverse aspects of health and vitality, from its potential role in managing metabolic health to its influence on energy levels, mental clarity, and overall vitality. Through evidence-based insights and real-world testimonials, readers will gain a holistic perspective on the far-reaching benefits of embracing the Dukan Diet as a transformative lifestyle choice.

As you turn the pages, envision a life where your relationship with food transforms, where weight loss is not a destination but a sustainable journey. The benefits awaiting you are not merely physical; they are the keys to unlocking a renewed sense of self. Welcome to a narrative where your well-being takes center stage, and the benefits are as profound as the journey itself. Get ready to immerse yourself in the transformative magic of the Dukan Diet.

CHAPTER 2

In-depth exploration of the four key phases of the Dukan Diet – Attack, Cruise, Consolidation, and Stabilization.

In the upcoming chapters, readers will embark on an in-depth exploration of the four key phases that form the foundation of the Dukan Diet – the Attack, Cruise, Consolidation, and Stabilization phases. This comprehensive journey will unravel the intricacies, rationale, and transformative potential of each phase, equipping readers with a profound understanding of how this structured approach can revolutionize their relationship with food, weight management, and overall well-being.

The Attack phase, renowned for its rapid initial weight loss results, will be dissected to reveal the science behind its emphasis on lean protein consumption and its potential to kickstart the body's fat burning mechanisms. Readers will gain insight into the strategic duration and dietary guidelines of this phase, empowering them to harness its transformative potential as a catalyst for sustainable weight loss and metabolic recalibration.

Moving forward, the Cruise phase will be unveiled as a pivotal bridge to long-term success, offering a balanced approach to sustained weight loss through the alternating rhythm of lean protein days and vegetable days. Journey into an intense, high-impact initiation designed to kickstart your weight loss. Explore the science behind this protein-rich phase and learn how it transforms your body into a fat-burning furnace. Readers will uncover the science behind this phase's metabolic optimization and its potential to cultivate a balanced, sustainable approach to weight management that transcends quick fixes and fad diets. As we set sail into the Cruise Phase, discover the art of balancing lean proteins and select vegetables. Uncover the secrets of culinary creativity, turning your kitchen into a haven of healthy, delicious meals. This phase isn't just a continuation; it's a voyage into a world where flavor and nutrition coexist.

The Consolidation phase will emerge as a transformative juncture, where readers will gain a nuanced understanding of the dietary and lifestyle principles that underpin its role in fortifying weight loss, restoring metabolic equilibrium, and nurturing a sustainable relationship with food. This phase's emphasis on gradual reintroduction of diverse food groups and its potential to recalibrate the body's response to dietary choices will be illuminated with practical insights and evidence-based guidance. The Consolidation Phase isn't just a transition; it's the foundation upon which lasting success is built. Delve into the gradual reintroduction of foods, the protective shield against the rebound effect, and the cultivation of habits that will endure beyond the diet.

Finally, the Stabilization phase will be unveiled as the cornerstone of long-term success, empowering readers to cultivate a sustainable, balanced approach to weight management and overall well-being. By unraveling the principles of this phase's enduring guidelines, readers will gain a comprehensive understanding of how to harness the transformative potential of the Dukan Diet as a lifelong strategy for vitality, metabolic health, and holistic well-being. The journey doesn't end; it evolves into the lifelong commitment of the Stabilization Phase. Explore how the principles learned in the preceding phases seamlessly integrate into a balanced, sustainable lifestyle. This isn't just about maintaining weight; it's about embracing a future of wellness.

Through this in-depth exploration of the four key phases of the Dukan Diet, readers will emerge with a profound understanding of the diet's transformative potential, empowering them to embark on a sustainable, personalized journey towards a healthier, more vibrant future. Brace yourself for an extraordinary odyssey through the meticulously structured landscape of the Dukan Diet, where each phase holds the potential to ignite a beacon of hope and inspiration for a transformative relationship with food and well-being.

Understanding the purpose and methodology of each phase for maximum weight loss and sustainable results

In the upcoming chapters, readers will embark on a captivating exploration of the purpose and methodology behind each phase of the Dukan Diet, unveiling a comprehensive understanding of how this structured approach fosters maximum weight loss and sustainable results. This transformative journey will offer a multifaceted perspective on the strategic rationale and scientific underpinnings of each phase, empowering readers to embrace a holistic, evidence-based approach to their own wellness journey.

The purpose and methodology of the Attack phase will be illuminated, offering readers a profound understanding of its role as a catalyst for rapid weight loss and metabolic recalibration. By unraveling the science behind its strategic emphasis on lean protein consumption and its potential to ignite the body's fat-burning machinery, readers will gain a comprehensive understanding of how this phase sets the stage for sustainable results and a transformative relationship with food and vitality.

Moving forward, the methodology and transformative potential of the Cruise phase will be unveiled, offering readers a captivating perspective on its balanced approach to sustained weight loss through the alternating rhythm of lean protein days and vegetable days. By illuminating the science behind this phase's metabolic optimization and its potential to cultivate a balanced, sustainable approach to weight management, readers will gain empowerment and insight to navigate this pivotal leg of their journey with confidence and resilience.

Furthermore, the purpose and methodology of the Consolidation and Stabilization phases will emerge as transformative junctures, offering readers a nuanced understanding of their roles in fortifying weight loss, restoring metabolic equilibrium, and nurturing a sustainable relationship with food. Through evidence-based insights and practical guidance, readers will gain a comprehensive understanding of how these phases lay the groundwork for long-term success and a redefined approach to holistic well-being.

Ultimately, this captivating exploration of the purpose and methodology behind each phase of the Dukan Diet will equip readers with a profound understanding of how this structured approach catalyzes maximum weight loss and sustainable results. Get ready to embark on an extraordinary odyssey through the transformative landscape of the Dukan Diet's phases, where each revelation holds the potential to ignite a beacon of hope and inspiration for a healthier, more vibrant future.

CHAPTER 3

The Attack Phase

The Attack Phase of the Dukan Diet is designed to kickstart weight loss by facilitating rapid fat burning and metabolic recalibration. This initial phase typically lasts between 2 to 7 days, depending on an individual's weight loss goals and starting weight. The primary focus of this phase is on consuming high-protein foods while strictly limiting carbohydrates and fats. This strategic dietary approach is aimed at inducing a state of ketosis, where the body shifts from using carbohydrates for energy to burning stored fat.

During the Attack Phase, individuals are encouraged to consume lean proteins such as skinless poultry, fish, lean cuts of beef or pork, tofu, and low-fat dairy products. These protein sources are not only satiating but also require the body to expend more energy for digestion, thereby boosting the metabolic rate. The absence of carbohydrates and fats during this phase prompts the body to tap into its fat stores for fuel, leading to rapid weight loss.

By focusing on protein-rich foods, individuals can experience reduced feelings of hunger and cravings, which are common barriers to adhering to a weight loss plan. The Attack Phase can often result in significant initial weight loss, making it an encouraging and motivating start to the Dukan Diet journey.

It's important to note that while the Attack Phase is effective for jumpstarting weight loss, it is just the beginning of a longer-term lifestyle change. The subsequent phases of the Dukan Diet, such as the Cruise, Consolidation, and Stabilization phases, are essential for achieving sustainable results and maintaining a healthy weight in the long run.

As we dissect this transformative phase, you'll gain a comprehensive understanding of the science, purpose, and methodology that make the Attack Phase the cornerstone of your Dukan journey.

1. Purpose: Igniting the Metabolic Furnace

   - The Attack Phase serves as the metabolism's wake-up call. Explore how the exclusive focus on lean proteins jumpstarts the fat-burning process, initiating swift weight loss.

   - Gain insight into the physiological changes that occur during this phase, understanding how the body shifts from using carbohydrates to tapping into its fat reserves for energy.

2. Methodology: The Protein Powerhouse

- Dive into the world of proteins as the primary fuel source. Understand why lean meats, poultry, fish, eggs, and non-fat dairy become the protagonists of your dietary choices.

- Uncover the strategic role of protein in inducing a feeling of fullness, reducing cravings, and preserving muscle mass—a crucial element for sustained weight loss

3. Duration and Transition: Navigating the Onset

- Understand the recommended duration of the Attack Phase and how it varies based on individual weight loss goals.

- Gain insights into the smooth transition from the Attack Phase to the subsequent stages, ensuring a seamless progression through the Dukan Diet.

4. Monitoring Progress: The Role of Measurement

- Explore the importance of monitoring progress during the Attack Phase. Discuss tools such as weight measurements, body fat percentage assessments, and other indicators of success.

- Learn to differentiate between short-term water weight loss and sustainable fat loss, setting realistic expectations for the transformative journey ahead.

Strategies for kickstarting weight loss with a focus on lean proteins

Kickstarting weight loss with a focus on lean proteins involves strategic dietary and lifestyle choices that harness the thermogenic and satiating properties of protein to fuel fat burning and enhance metabolic efficiency. Here are some effective strategies for leveraging lean proteins to initiate and sustain weight loss:

1. Embracing Protein-Dense Foods: Incorporate a variety of lean protein sources into your meals, including skinless poultry, fish, lean cuts of beef or pork, tofu, legumes, and low-fat dairy products. These foods not only provide essential nutrients but also contribute to a feeling of fullness, reducing the likelihood of overeating.

2. Balancing Macronutrients: While emphasizing lean proteins, it's important to strike a balance with healthy fats and complex carbohydrates. Opt for sources of healthy fats such as avocados, nuts, and olive oil, and include complex carbohydrates from vegetables, fruits, and whole grains. This balanced approach supports overall nutritional needs and promotes sustainable weight loss.

3. Prioritizing Whole Foods: Choose whole, minimally processed foods to maximize the nutritional benefits of lean proteins. Avoid highly processed or fried protein sources, as they may contain added fats and unhealthy additives that can hinder weight loss efforts.

4. Portion Control and Timing: Be mindful of portion sizes when consuming lean proteins, and aim to distribute protein intake evenly across meals and snacks throughout the day. This strategic approach can help regulate appetite, stabilize blood sugar levels, and optimize metabolism.

5. Incorporating Resistance Training: Pairing a protein-rich diet with regular resistance training can further enhance the body's ability to build and maintain lean muscle mass. Muscle tissue has a higher metabolic rate than fat, so increasing muscle mass can contribute to a more efficient metabolism and greater calorie expenditure, aiding in weight loss efforts.

6. Hydration and Fiber: Support your protein-focused diet with adequate hydration and fiber intake. Water and fiber-rich foods

can enhance digestion, promote satiety, and support overall metabolic function, complementing the effects of lean proteins on weight loss.

By incorporating these strategies, the focus on lean proteins during the Attack Phase becomes not just a dietary guideline but a personalized and sustainable approach to kickstarting your weight loss journey. Welcome to a chapter where the strategic alliance between your choices and the principles of the Dukan Diet sets the stage for transformative success.

Navigating Challenges and Staying Motivated in the Attack Phase

The initial phase of a weight loss journey, particularly when focusing on lean proteins, can present unique challenges. However, with practical tips and strategies, individuals can overcome these hurdles and stay motivated during this crucial phase:

1. Meal Planning and Preparation: Invest time in planning and preparing meals that are rich in lean proteins. Having pre-portioned, protein-packed meals readily available can help avoid impulsive, less healthy food choices.

2. Diversifying Protein Sources: Explore a variety of lean protein options to prevent culinary monotony. Experiment with different cooking methods and flavor profiles to keep meals interesting and enjoyable.

3. Seeking Support and Accountability: Engage with a support system, whether it's a friend, family member, or online community, to share experiences and receive encouragement. Accountability partners can offer motivation and help navigate challenges.

4. Setting Realistic Goals: Establish achievable short-term and long-term goals related to weight loss and overall wellness. Celebrate small victories along the way and maintain a positive mindset.

5. Incorporating Flavorful Seasonings: Enhance the taste of lean proteins with herbs, spices, and healthy condiments. This can make meals more satisfying and enjoyable, mitigating the perception of dietary restrictions.

6. Mindful Eating Practices: Practice mindful eating by savoring each bite and paying attention to hunger and fullness cues. This can prevent overeating and foster a more conscious relationship with food.

7. Physical Activity and Movement: Engage in regular physical activity, such as brisk walking, yoga, or strength training. Exercise not only supports weight loss but also enhances overall well-being and can boost motivation.

8. Flexibility and Adaptability: Be flexible and open to adjustments in the dietary approach. If a particular protein source becomes monotonous, explore new options and recipes to maintain enthusiasm.

9. Tracking Progress: Keep a journal to track dietary choices, physical activity, and emotional well-being. Reflecting on progress and challenges can provide valuable insights and motivation.

10. Self-compassion and Patience: Practice self-compassion and patience, recognizing that sustainable weight loss is a gradual process. Embrace setbacks as learning opportunities and stay committed to the journey.

By integrating these practical tips into the weight loss journey, individuals can navigate the challenges of focusing on lean proteins and stay motivated during this crucial phase, ultimately setting the stage for successful and sustainable progress.

CHAPTER 4

The cruise phase

Transitioning from a pure protein-focused phase to a phase that incorporates both protein and vegetables is a pivotal juncture in the weight loss journey, signifying a shift towards a more balanced and sustainable approach to nutrition. Navigating this transition effectively requires a thoughtful and informed strategy to maintain momentum and optimize progress. Here are key considerations and practical tips for successfully transitioning from a pure protein phase to one that embraces protein and vegetable combinations:

<u>Gradual Introduction</u>: Introduce vegetables gradually as you transition from a pure protein phase. Begin by incorporating non-starchy vegetables such as leafy greens, cucumbers, tomatoes, and bell peppers, which are low in carbohydrates and can complement lean proteins effectively.

<u>Portion Control</u>: Pay attention to portion sizes when adding vegetables to meals. Balancing protein and vegetables ensures that the meal remains satiating and supports the body's nutritional needs while promoting weight loss.

<u>Nutrient Diversity</u>: Embrace a diverse array of vegetables to benefit from their varied nutrients, vitamins, and antioxidants. Aim to include a spectrum of colors and textures in your vegetable choices to maximize nutritional intake.

Strategic Pairing: Pairing lean proteins with fiber-rich vegetables can enhance satiety and promote digestive health. This combination can also contribute to a more balanced and sustainable approach to weight management.

Meal Planning: Plan meals that incorporate a balance of lean proteins and vegetables. Adopting a structured meal plan can help ensure that both food groups are included in a way that supports weight loss and overall well-being.

Experimenting with Cooking Methods: Explore diverse cooking methods for vegetables, such as steaming, roasting, or stir-frying, to enhance their flavors and textures. Experimenting with different culinary techniques can make the transition more enjoyable and sustainable.

Hydration and Fiber: As vegetables are introduced, ensure adequate hydration and fiber intake to support digestion and satiety. Hydrating vegetables, such as cucumbers and celery, can contribute to overall fluid intake and aid in the feeling of fullness.

Mindful Eating: Practice mindful eating by savoring the combination of lean proteins and vegetables. Pay attention to the flavors, textures, and nourishing qualities of each meal to cultivate a more conscious and positive relationship with food.

Flexibility and Adaptability: Be open to adjusting the types and quantities of vegetables based on personal preferences and nutritional needs. Flexibility allows for a more sustainable and enjoyable dietary transition.

As you embark on the Cruise Phase, envision it as a culinary odyssey — a chapter where flavors intertwine, and nutritional variety becomes the cornerstone of your Dukan Diet journey. Welcome to a seamless transition where protein and vegetable combinations pave the way for a balanced and enjoyable approach to long-term well-being.

Navigating the transition from pure protein to protein and vegetable combinations.

Transitioning from a pure protein-focused phase to a phase that incorporates both protein and vegetables is a pivotal juncture in the weight loss journey, signifying a shift towards a more balanced and sustainable approach to nutrition. Navigating this transition effectively requires a thoughtful and informed strategy to maintain momentum and optimize progress. Here are key considerations and practical tips for successfully transitioning from a pure protein phase to one that embraces protein and vegetable combinations:

1. Understanding the Cruise Phase Transition:

- Explore the rationale behind transitioning from pure protein to protein and vegetable combinations. Understand how this shift introduces essential nutrients from vegetables while maintaining the protein-centric foundation established in the Attack Phase.

2. Gradual Introduction of Vegetables:

- Ease into the inclusion of vegetables by introducing them gradually. Start with those allowed in the Cruise Phase, such as leafy greens, cruciferous vegetables, and those with low starch content. This measured approach allows your body to adapt to the expanded menu.

3. Alternate Protein and Vegetable Days:

   - Embrace the alternating rhythm of protein and vegetable days. This structured approach not only adds variety to your meals but also ensures a balanced intake over the course of the Cruise Phase.

4. Crafting Balanced Meals:

   - Explore the art of crafting balanced meals that blend proteins and vegetables in appealing combinations. Experiment with different cooking techniques, herbs, and spices to enhance flavor and maintain the nutritional integrity of each dish.

5. Explore New Culinary Horizons:

   - View the Cruise Phase as an opportunity to expand your culinary horizons. Experiment with diverse vegetables and protein sources to keep your meals exciting and satisfying. This phase is not just a transition; it's a voyage into the joy of wholesome eating.

6. Monitoring Progress:

   - Continue to monitor your progress during the Cruise Phase. Pay attention to how your body responds to the introduction of vegetables, and adjust your approach based on your individual needs and goals.

7. Mindful Eating Practices:

   - Practice mindful eating as you navigate the combination of proteins and vegetables. Pay attention to portion sizes, savor the flavors of each component, and cultivate a deeper connection with the act of eating.

8. Addressing Challenges Proactively:

   - Anticipate and address challenges that may arise during the transition. Whether it's adapting to new flavors or managing the temptation of less restrictive options, proactively addressing challenges enhances your success in the Cruise Phase.

9. Celebrate Culinary Creativity:

- Celebrate the creativity that comes with combining proteins and vegetables. The Cruise Phase isn't just about nutritional variety; it's an invitation to revel in the pleasure of diverse and delicious meals.

10. Consult with a Nutrition Professional:

- Consider consulting with a nutrition professional for personalized guidance. They can offer tailored advice on crafting balanced meals, meeting nutritional requirements, and optimizing your approach to the Cruise Phase.

By embracing these strategies and considerations, individuals can navigate the transition from a pure protein phase to one that incorporates protein and vegetable combinations with confidence and success, setting the stage for continued progress and sustainable weight management.

Crafting a balanced and satisfying menu during the Cruise Phase

The Cruise Phase of the Dukan Diet introduces a balanced approach by incorporating both protein and vegetables, offering a wider variety of food choices while supporting continued weight loss. Crafting a balanced and satisfying menu during this phase involves strategic meal planning and the thoughtful combination of lean proteins and an array of vegetables. Here's a sample menu that exemplifies the principles of the Cruise Phase:

Breakfast:

- Omelette made with egg whites, diced lean ham, and a variety of colorful vegetables such as spinach, bell peppers, and tomatoes

- A side of low-fat Greek yogurt topped with fresh berries

- Herbal tea or black coffee

Mid-Morning Snack:

- A protein-rich snack, such as a serving of low-fat cottage cheese or a hard-boiled egg

- A small serving of raw, crunchy vegetables like cucumber slices or celery sticks

Lunch:

- Grilled chicken breast or fish fillet seasoned with herbs and lemon juice

- A generous mixed salad featuring lettuce, arugula, cucumbers, cherry tomatoes, and radishes

- A light vinaigrette made with balsamic vinegar and a touch of olive oil

- A side of steamed broccoli or asparagus

Afternoon Snack:

- A protein-packed snack, such as turkey slices or a serving of low-fat string cheese

- A small portion of raw vegetables, such as carrot sticks or cherry tomatoes

Dinner:

- Lean beef or tofu stir-fry with an assortment of colorful bell peppers, snap peas, and onions

- A side of steamed cauliflower or zucchini

- A light and refreshing cucumber and dill salad dressed with low-fat yogurt

- A cup of herbal tea or infused water

Evening Snack:

- A small serving of low-fat yogurt topped with a sprinkle of chia seeds or sliced almonds

- A portion of fresh berries or a citrus fruit

Incorporating this menu into the Cruise Phase embraces a balanced combination of lean proteins and an assortment of nutrient-rich vegetables, providing a satisfying and varied array of flavors and textures. This approach supports ongoing weight loss while promoting satiety and overall nutritional well-being.

It's important to customize this menu to individual tastes and dietary needs, while ensuring that the principles of the Cruise Phase, which emphasize protein and vegetable combinations, are upheld. Additionally, staying hydrated by consuming an adequate amount of water throughout the day is essential for overall health and weight management during this phase.

CHAPTER 5

The Consolidation Phase Unveiled

The Consolidation Phase of the Dukan Diet marks a crucial transition towards long-term weight maintenance and the cultivation of sustainable eating habits. This phase is designed to solidify the achievements of the previous phases while gradually reintroducing a wider variety of foods into the diet. The primary goals of the Consolidation Phase include preventing the rapid regain of lost weight, promoting metabolic stability, and nurturing a balanced and healthy relationship with food. As you progress through the transformative journey of the Dukan Diet, the Consolidation Phase emerges as a pivotal chapter—a bridge from weight loss achievements to enduring well-being. In this chapter, we delve into the essence of the Consolidation Phase, understanding its purpose, methodology, and the foundational principles that fortify your progress.

1. The Significance of Consolidation:

   - Uncover the critical role the Consolidation Phase plays in safeguarding your weight loss achievements. This phase is not just a transition; it's the consolidation of your newfound well-being, ensuring resilience against the rebound effect.

2. Preventing the Rebound Effect:

   - Explore how the Consolidation Phase acts as a protective shield, preventing the all-too-common rebound effect associated with many weight loss regimens. Understand the science behind gradually reintroducing certain foods, fostering sustainability without compromising progress.

3. Gradual Reintroduction of Foods:

- Delve into the strategic reintroduction of previously restricted foods. Learn how this gradual process, guided by clear rules, balances variety and nutritional intake while minimizing the risk of regaining lost weight.

4. Celebratory Meals and Milestones:

- Embrace the concept of celebratory meals and milestones during the Consolidation Phase. Discover how these moments are not just culinary indulgences but integral to reinforcing your accomplishments and fostering a positive relationship with food.

5. Building Habits for Lifelong Success:

- Navigate the establishment of habits during the Consolidation Phase that will endure beyond the Dukan Diet. Understand how these habits, centered around balanced nutrition and mindful eating, become the foundation for lifelong well-being.

6. Tailoring Consolidation to Your Journey:

- Recognize the flexibility within the Consolidation Phase, allowing for tailoring to individual needs and experiences. Whether you're continuing weight loss or focusing on weight maintenance, the Consolidation Phase adapts to your unique journey.

7. Monitoring Progress and Adjusting:

- Discover the importance of ongoing progress monitoring during the Consolidation Phase. Learn to assess your achievements, make adjustments as needed, and cultivate a proactive approach to maintaining your well-being.

8. Transitioning to Stabilization:

   - Gain insights into the seamless transition from the Consolidation Phase to the lifelong commitment of the Stabilization Phase. Understand how the habits cultivated during consolidation become the building blocks for a future of balanced living.

As you immerse yourself in the Consolidation Phase, envision it not just as a stage in your journey but as a transformative period laying the groundwork for a resilient and balanced future. Welcome to a chapter where consolidation becomes synonymous with lasting success, and your progress is fortified for the horizons ahead.

Concept of mindful eatings in this phase

Mindful eating is a fundamental concept that holds significant importance, especially during the Consolidation Phase of the Dukan Diet. This phase emphasizes the cultivation of a balanced and sustainable relationship with food, promoting mindfulness, awareness, and a positive approach to eating. Here's an in-depth exploration of the concept of mindful eating in the context of the Consolidation Phase:

1. Present-Moment Awareness: Mindful eating involves being fully present and engaged in the act of eating, focusing on the sensory experience of each bite. This includes paying attention to the taste, texture, aroma, and visual appeal of food.

2. Appreciation of Food: Mindful eating encourages individuals to develop a deeper appreciation for the nourishing qualities of food, fostering gratitude for the sustenance and pleasure that meals provide.

3. Conscious Portion Control: By practicing mindful eating, individuals can become more attuned to their body's hunger and satiety signals, leading to more conscious portion control and a reduced likelihood of overeating.

4. Emotional Awareness: Mindful eating involves recognizing and acknowledging emotional cues related to food, such as stress eating or eating out of boredom. This awareness enables individuals to develop healthier coping strategies and a more balanced relationship with food.

5. Savoring the Experience: Mindful eating emphasizes the importance of savoring each bite, allowing individuals to derive greater satisfaction from their meals and fostering a more pleasurable and fulfilling eating experience.

6. Connection to Nutritional Choices: Engaging in mindful eating encourages individuals to consider the nutritional value of their food choices, promoting the selection of nourishing, whole foods that support overall well-being and health.

7. Slower, More Deliberate Eating: Mindful eating involves slowing down the pace of eating and taking the time to chew food thoroughly, which can enhance digestion, promote satiety, and contribute to a more mindful and enjoyable meal experience.

8. Reduction of Distractions: Practicing mindful eating often involves minimizing distractions during meals, such as electronic devices or multitasking, allowing individuals to focus solely on the act of eating and the enjoyment of their food.

Examples of mindful eating practices

Mindful eating practices plays a pivotal role in promoting a balanced and sustainable approach to nutrition during the Consolidation Phase of the Dukan Diet. Here, some specific examples of mindful eating practices individuals can incorporate during this phase:

1. Sensory Exploration: Prior to taking the first bite, take a moment to visually appreciate the colors and presentation of the meal. Notice the aroma of the food and acknowledge the anticipation of the flavors to come. This sensory exploration cultivates

a heightened awareness and appreciation for the meal.

2. <u>Portion Awareness</u>: Pay attention to portion sizes and serving sizes, using visual cues and mindful observation to gauge an appropriate amount of food. This practice supports conscious portion control and encourages eating in alignment with individual nutritional needs.

3. <u>Slow and Deliberate Eating</u>: Practice eating at a slower pace, taking the time to chew each bite thoroughly and savor the flavors and textures of the food. By slowing down the eating process, individuals can enhance digestion, promote satiety, and foster a more mindful and enjoyable meal experience.

4. <u>Mindful Snacking</u>: When incorporating snacks into the day, approach them with mindfulness. Take the time to acknowledge hunger cues, choose nutritious snack options, and savor the experience of eating, even during snack times. This practice supports balanced energy levels and prevents mindless snacking.

5. <u>Gratitude and Appreciation</u>: Before starting a meal, take a moment to express gratitude for the nourishing qualities of the food and the effort that went into its preparation. Cultivating a sense of appreciation for the meal can enhance the overall enjoyment of eating and foster a positive relationship with food.

6. <u>Emotionally Attuned Eating</u>: Pay attention to emotional cues related to food choices and eating habits. Acknowledge the

connection between emotions and eating behaviors, practicing mindfulness to differentiate between physical hunger and emotional triggers for eating.

7. <u>Distraction-Free Dining</u>: By creating an environment conducive to mindful eating by minimizing distractions during meals. Turn off electronic devices, set aside work-related activities, and focus solely on the act of eating and the experience of enjoying the meal.

8. <u>Reflective Eating</u>: After completing a meal, take a moment to reflect on the experience. Notice how the food made you feel physically and emotionally, and consider the ways in which mindful eating practices have enhanced your mealtime experience.

By integrating these mindful eating practices into the Consolidation Phase, individuals can cultivate a more balanced and sustainable approach to nutrition, fostering a deeper connection to the act of eating and the nourishing qualities of food. These practices align with the overarching goals of the Consolidation Phase, supporting long-term success in weight maintenance and overall well-being.

Preventing the rebound effect

By methodically reintroducing select foods, promoting a balanced approach to nutrition, and mitigating the potential rebound effect after weight loss, this phase will fortify your progress while indulging in a diverse array of delectable sustenance.

Gradual Reintroduction of Foods: Striking the Perfect Balance

During the Consolidation Phase, we adopt a meticulously gradual approach to reintegrate foods that were previously restricted. This calculated strategy effectively prevents your body from succumbing to the perils of "starvation mode" and safeguards against a decelerated metabolism. By systematically incorporating fruits, starchy foods, and selected fats, we facilitate your body's seamless adaptation to a broader spectrum of vital nutrients, ensuring an optimally functioning metabolism.

Here are some examples of foods that are reintroduced during this phase:

- Fruits: One serving of fruit per day is initially reintroduced, excluding bananas, grapes, figs, and cherries. In the second half of the Consolidation Phase, this increases to two servings of fruit per day.

- Whole Grain Bread: During the first half of the Consolidation Phase, two slices of whole grain bread per day are added to the diet and this remains the same in the second half as well.

- Hard Rind Cheese: In the Consolidation Phase, 5 ounces of hard rind cheese are introduced into the diet.

- Starchy Foods: In the first half of the Consolidation Phase, one serving (cooked cup) of starchy foods is reintroduced every week. In the second half, this increases to two servings (cooked cup) of starchy foods per week.

- Celebration Meals: Initially, one celebration meal per week is allowed, which includes 1 appetizer, 1 entrée, 1 dessert, and 1 glass of wine. In the later part of the phase, this increases to two celebration meals per week.

These gradual reintroductions are part of the structured approach of the Consolidation Phase to transition from a more restrictive diet to a more varied and balanced eating plan while aiming to prevent rebound weight gain.

Stabilizing Metabolic Rate: Nurturing Your Body's Equilibrium

Our primary concern is to maintain a stable metabolic rate that doesn't plummet unexpectedly, as this can impede your ability to sustain weight loss. Through the gradual increment of caloric intake and the diversification of your culinary choices, we empower your body to remain resilient and prevent acclimatization to lower calorie thresholds. This comprehensive approach enables you to savor an expanded repertoire of foods without the distressing prospect of swift weight regain.

Sustainable Eating Habits: Forging a Lifelong Commitment to Health

The Consolidation Phase is unequivocally dedicated to instilling sustainable eating habits that can endure the test of time. We advocate for portion control, judicious food selection, and mindful consumption practices, paving the way for a harmonious equilibrium that suits your unique needs. By focusing on sustainable changes rather than fleeting restrictions, we lay the groundwork for enduring success in maintaining your weight loss accomplishments, all while ensuring that you never feel deprived.

Psychological Satisfaction and Moderation: Prioritizing Your Well-Being

We acknowledge the profound significance of psychological satisfaction and the enjoyment of the foods you hold dear. To that end, we introduce "celebration meals" and foster a spirit of moderation during this phase. By incorporating occasional indulgences and promoting a measured approach, we grant you the freedom to revel in your culinary desires without succumbing to the temptation to overcompensate after periods of stringent dieting. Our aim is to facilitate a delicate balance that nourishes not only your body but your mind as well.

Long-Term Support and Guidance: We're Your Trusted Allies

We firmly believe in providing unwavering support and unyielding guidance to ensure your unwavering motivation and sustainable decision-making. Our dedicated team remains committed to being your steadfast companion throughout your weight loss journey and beyond. We understand that having a dependable ally by your side can make all the difference in maintaining your progress and safeguarding your overall well-being.

In conclusion, the Consolidation Phase of the Dukan Diet serves as an authoritative blueprint that propels you towards long-term success. By meticulously reintroducing foods, stabilizing your metabolic rate, fostering sustainable eating habits, encouraging psychological satisfaction and moderation, and offering ongoing support and guidance, we are honored to play a pivotal role in your pursuit of a healthier and more fulfilling life. Our team is always here to provide you with the support and guidance you need on your journey. Remember, you are not alone, and together we can achieve the long-term success you desire.

CHAPTER 6

The stabilization phase

The Stabilization Phase is the crowning jewel of the Dukan Diet, representing the transition from active weight loss to a sustainable and balanced lifestyle. This phase is designed to consolidate your achievements, fortify new habits, and guide you towards lifelong well-being.

Transitioning into the Lifelong Stabilization Phase of the Dukan Diet marks a significant milestone in your journey towards sustainable weight management and overall well-being. This phase, designed to be a permanent lifestyle approach, focuses on maintaining the achievements of the previous phases while embracing a balanced and varied diet. Here's a guide to help you understand the key principles and strategies for a successful transition into the Lifelong Stabilization Phase:

Embracing Lasting Habits

As you transition into the Lifelong Stabilization Phase, it's crucial to internalize the healthy habits and practices developed during the earlier phases of the Dukan Diet. These include portion control, mindful eating, and making informed food choices. By embracing these lasting habits, you'll lay a solid foundation for sustaining your progress in the long term.

Balancing Nutritional Variety

The Lifelong Stabilization Phase encourages a balanced and varied diet that includes a wide range of nutrient-dense foods. It's essential to incorporate lean proteins, healthy fats, fiber-rich carbohydrates, and an ample supply of fruits and vegetables into your daily meals. This balanced nutritional approach not only supports weight maintenance but also contributes to overall health and vitality.

Moderating Celebratory Indulgences

While the Lifelong Stabilization Phase allows for occasional indulgences, it's important to practice moderation when enjoying celebratory meals and special treats. By incorporating these indulgences mindfully and in moderation, you can savor your favorite foods without compromising your long-term progress.

Prioritizing Physical Activity

Regular physical activity remains a cornerstone of the Lifelong Stabilization Phase. Engaging in a mix of cardiovascular exercises, strength training, and other physical activities not only supports weight maintenance but also promotes overall fitness, strength, and well-being.

Cultivating a Supportive Environment

Transitioning into the Lifelong Stabilization Phase may benefit from the support of friends, family, or fellow Dukan Diet participants. By fostering a supportive environment, you can stay motivated, share experiences, and continue to make healthy choices as part of a community dedicated to long-term well-being.

Monitoring Your Progress

Regular self-monitoring, such as weighing yourself weekly and reflecting on your eating and exercise habits, can be beneficial during the Lifelong Stabilization Phase. It allows you to stay mindful of your progress and make adjustments as needed to maintain your desired weight and overall health.

Seeking Professional Guidance

For personalized support and guidance during the transition into the Lifelong Stabilization Phase, consider consulting with a registered dietitian, nutritionist, or healthcare professional. Their expertise can help tailor your eating plan to suit your individual needs and ensure that you continue to make informed choices for sustained success.

Celebrating Achievements

Finally, transitioning into the Lifelong Stabilization Phase presents an opportunity to celebrate your achievements and the progress you've made throughout your Dukan Diet journey. Recognizing and celebrating your success can reinforce your commitment to a healthier lifestyle and motivate you to maintain your newfound sense of well-being.

In essence, transitioning into the Lifelong Stabilization Phase is about integrating the principles of the Dukan Diet into a sustainable, balanced, and enjoyable way of life. By embracing healthy habits, balancing nutritional variety, practicing moderation, prioritizing physical activity, cultivating support, monitoring progress, seeking professional guidance, and celebrating achievements, you can confidently embark on this lifelong phase with a focus on sustained success and well-being.

Strategies for Weight Maintenance and a Balanced Lifestyle

Congratulations on reaching the point where maintaining your weight loss and embracing a balanced lifestyle become the focal points of your journey. In this chapter, we'll explore essential strategies that will not only help you sustain your success but also prevent relapse, ensuring that the achievements of the Dukan Diet endure in the long term.

1. Mindful Eating as a Lifelong Practice:

   - Cultivate mindful eating as a permanent practice. Pay attention to your body's hunger and fullness signals, savor the flavors of your meals, and be present in the eating experience. Mindful eating fosters a healthy relationship with food and prevents overindulgence.

- Pay attention to hunger and fullness cues, and eat slowly to savor and enjoy your meals.

- Be conscious of emotional eating triggers and find alternative coping strategies to manage emotions without turning to food.

2. Regular Physical Activity:

- Maintain a commitment to regular physical activity. Incorporate exercises that you enjoy into your routine, whether it's walking, jogging, cycling, or engaging in fitness classes. Physical activity not only supports weight maintenance but also contributes to overall well-being.

- Engage in regular exercise, including a mix of cardiovascular activities, strength training, and flexibility exercises.

- Aim for at least 150 minutes of moderate-intensity aerobic activity or 75 minutes of vigorous-intensity aerobic activity each week, along with muscle-strengthening activities on two or more days a week.

3. Balanced Nutrition as a Priority:

- Prioritize balanced nutrition by continuing to incorporate a variety of food groups into your meals. Ensure that your diet includes lean proteins, vegetables, fruits, whole grains, and healthy fats. This balanced approach provides essential nutrients for sustained health.

- Prioritize a balanced diet rich in fruits, vegetables, whole grains, lean proteins, and healthy fats.

- Practice portion control and mindful eating to maintain a healthy relationship with food and prevent overeating.

4. Set Realistic and Sustainable Goals:

   - Establish realistic and sustainable goals for yourself. Avoid setting targets that are too restrictive or demanding, as this can lead to frustration and a higher risk of relapse. Celebrate small victories and progress towards your long-term objectives.

5. Regular Monitoring and Adjustments:

   - Continue to monitor your progress regularly. This includes tracking your weight, assessing your fitness levels, and evaluating your overall well-being. Be proactive in making adjustments to your lifestyle, diet, or exercise routine as needed.

   - Weigh yourself regularly to track your progress and make adjustments if necessary.

- Keep a food diary to monitor your eating habits and identify any patterns that may need adjustment.

6. Stay Connected with Support Systems:

- Maintain connections with your support systems. Whether it's friends, family, or individuals who share similar health and wellness goals, having a support network can provide encouragement, motivation, and accountability.

7. Mindfulness in Food Choices:

- Be mindful of your food choices even when faced with occasional indulgences. Allow yourself treats in moderation and avoid an "all-or-nothing" mentality. Balancing enjoyment with nutritional consciousness is key to preventing feelings of deprivation.

8. Address Emotional Eating:

   - Recognize and address emotional eating patterns. Understand the triggers that may lead to emotional eating and develop healthy coping mechanisms. Strategies such as journaling, meditation, or seeking professional support can be beneficial.

9. Revisit and Reinforce Dukan Principles:

   - Revisit the fundamental principles of the Dukan Diet periodically. This can serve as a reminder of the habits and strategies that contributed to your success. Reinforcing these principles helps anchor your commitment to a balanced lifestyle.

By incorporating these strategies into your daily life, you are not only maintaining your weight loss but also embracing a holistic approach to well-being. Welcome to a chapter where success is not just a fleeting achievement but a sustainable and fulfilling way of life.

Preventing relapse

Preventing relapse and maintaining long-term success after completing a diet, such as the Dukan Diet, involves adopting sustainable lifestyle habits. Here are some tips to help prevent relapse:

1. Gradual Transition:

   - If you're transitioning out of a strict diet like the Dukan Diet, consider reintroducing forbidden foods gradually. Abruptly returning to old eating habits may lead to relapse.

2. Monitor Portion Sizes:

   - Be mindful of portion sizes to avoid overeating. Listen to your body's hunger cues, and try not to eat out of boredom.

3. Regular Exercise:

   - Incorporate regular physical activity into your routine. Exercise is not only beneficial for weight management but also for overall health and well-being.

 4. Balanced Nutrition:

   - Aim for a balanced diet that includes a variety of nutrient-dense foods. Ensure you are getting a mix of lean proteins, fruits, vegetables, whole grains, and healthy fats.

 5. Stay Hydrated:

   - Drink an adequate amount of water throughout the day. Sometimes, feelings of hunger can be mistaken for dehydration.

 6. Mindful Eating:

   - Practice mindful eating by savoring each bite, eating without distractions, and paying attention to hunger and fullness signals.

7. Regular Check-Ins:

   - Schedule regular check-ins with yourself to assess your eating habits and identify any potential challenges. Make adjustments as needed to stay on track.

8. Set Realistic Goals:

   - Set realistic and sustainable goals for yourself. Avoid extreme or restrictive diets that may lead to frustration and relapse.

9. Celebrate Non-Scale Victories:

   - Focus on more than just the number on the scale. Celebrate non-scale victories, such as increased energy, improved mood, or achieving fitness milestones.

10. Plan and Prep Meals:

   - Plan your meals in advance and prepare healthy options to have on hand. This can help you make nutritious choices, especially during busy or stressful times.

12. Manage Stress:

- Develop healthy stress management techniques, such as meditation, deep breathing exercises, or engaging in activities you enjoy. Stress can contribute to emotional eating.

13. Continuous Learning:

- Stay informed about nutrition and wellness. Continuous learning can empower you to make informed choices and understand the importance of a balanced and healthy lifestyle.

Remember that maintaining a healthy lifestyle is an ongoing process, and setbacks may happen. It's crucial to approach it with a mindset of progress, not perfection. If you find yourself struggling, seeking guidance from a healthcare professional or a registered dietitian can provide personalized support and strategies.

In "Book 2: Dukan Diet Recipes and Meal Plans," prepare to embark on a culinary journey that goes beyond sustenance—it's a celebration of flavors, creativity, and the continued success of your Dukan Diet lifestyle. Welcome to a book where each recipe is a chapter, and every meal is an opportunity to savor both nourishment and delight. Bon appétit!

A sneak peek into what readers can expect in "Book 2: Dukan Diet Recipes and Meal Plans" to continue their journey.

In "Book 2: Dukan Diet Recipes and Meal Plans," readers can expect an immersive and practical continuation of their journey with the Dukan Diet. This book offers a treasure trove of delectable recipes, customizable meal plans, and invaluable insights to support individuals in navigating the next phase of their wellness odyssey. Here's a sneak peek into what readers can expect:

1. Culinary Exploration:

- Discover an array of mouthwatering recipes tailored to the principles of the Dukan Diet, featuring diverse and flavorful dishes designed to tantalize the taste buds while aligning with your nutritional goals.

2. Customizable Meal Plans:

   - Access meticulously crafted meal plans that cater to various dietary preferences and lifestyle needs, providing a roadmap for seamlessly integrating the Dukan Diet into your daily routine.

3. Nutritional Guidance:

   - Gain deeper insights into the nutritional principles underpinning the Dukan Diet, empowering you to make informed choices and optimize your eating habits for sustained well-being.

4. Innovative Cooking Techniques:

   - Uncover innovative cooking techniques and culinary tips to elevate your meal preparation, ensuring that every dish is not only healthy but also a delight to create and savor.

5. Guidance for Adapting Recipes to Individual Preferences:

- Receive guidance on adapting recipes to individual preferences and dietary needs. Whether you have specific taste preferences, allergies, or cultural considerations, learn how to customize recipes without compromising the integrity of the Dukan Diet.

6. Supportive Resources:

- Access additional resources such as grocery shopping guides, pantry essentials, and practical tips for navigating social gatherings and travel while adhering to the Dukan Diet.

7. Success Stories and Testimonials:

- Draw inspiration from real-life success stories and testimonials from individuals who have embraced the Dukan Diet, providing a source of motivation and validation for your ongoing journey.

8. Wellness Beyond Food:

- Delve into holistic wellness practices, including fitness tips, stress management techniques, and strategies for nurturing a positive mindset, ensuring a comprehensive approach to your well-being.

9. Interactive Tools:

- Engage with interactive tools such as meal planning templates, recipe modification guidelines, and progress trackers to enrich your experience and facilitate your continued success.

10. Interactive Cooking Challenges and Tips:

- Engage in interactive cooking challenges and glean valuable tips from seasoned Dukan Diet enthusiasts. These challenges encourage experimentation, foster a sense of community, and enhance your culinary skills.

With "Book 2: Dukan Diet Recipes and Meal Plans," readers can anticipate a wealth of resources, inspiration, and guidance to propel them forward on their journey, ensuring that the principles of the Dukan Diet seamlessly integrate into their lives, ultimately leading to sustained well-being and vitality.

BONUS!! Sample recipe

Here's a sample recipe from the Dukan Diet for the Attack Phase:

Breakfast: Fried Eggs with Sliced Ham

Ingredients: Eggs, Sliced ham

Instructions:

 - Heat a non-stick pan over medium heat.

 - Add the sliced ham to the pan and cook until slightly browned.

 - Crack the eggs into the pan and cook to your desired level of doneness.

 - Serve the fried eggs with the sliced ham.

This simple and protein-rich breakfast option aligns with the guidelines of the Attack Phase of the Dukan Diet, providing a satisfying and nutritious start to the day.

Lunch Recipe - Tuna Patties

Ingredients: Canned tuna, Egg, Minced onion, Dijon mustard, Garlic powder, Black pepper, Salt, and olive oil for cooking

- Instructions:

1. In a bowl, combine canned tuna, beaten egg, minced onion, Dijon mustard, garlic powder, black pepper, and salt.

2. Form the mixture into patties.

3. Heat olive oil in a skillet over medium heat.

4. Cook the tuna patties until golden brown on each side.

5. Serve hot with a side of nonstarchy vegetables for a balanced n satisfying lunch.

This protein-packed recipe aligns with the guidelines of the Cruise Phase, offering a delicious and nutritious option for a well-rounded meal.

CONCLUSION

In conclusion, the "Dukan Diet Essentials" stands as a cornerstone of knowledge and empowerment in your quest for sustainable weight management and enhanced well-being. Through a comprehensive exploration of the Dukan Diet's core tenets, this book has equipped you with the essential understanding and tools to embark on a transformative journey toward a healthier lifestyle.

By delving into the fundamental principles of the Dukan Diet, you have gained insights into the importance of lean protein, non-starchy vegetables, healthy eating habits, and the phased approach that underpins this renowned dietary strategy. Armed with this knowledge, you are poised to embrace a balanced and healthful relationship with food, fostering a sustainable foundation for long-term success.

As you reflect on the wisdom imparted within these pages, may you find yourself empowered to make informed choices, cultivate mindful eating habits, and embark on a journey of holistic wellness. "Book 1" serves as a springboard for your ongoing pursuit of health, offering clarity, guidance, and the assurance that you are equipped with the knowledge needed to navigate the path ahead with confidence and purpose.

Let the principles outlined in this book be your compass, guiding you toward a lifestyle that harmonizes nourishment, well-being, and the fulfillment of your health goals. May your journey be marked by resilience, joy, and the transformative power of embracing the principles of the Dukan Diet as a catalyst for sustained vitality and healthy living.

It's not just the end of a chapter but the commencement of a transformative journey towards a healthier, more vibrant you. Throughout these pages, we've explored the principles, phases, and strategies that define the Dukan Diet—a path proven to lead to sustainable weight loss and lasting well-being.

In the pages that unfolded, you've gained insights into the four key phases— Attack, Cruise, Consolidation, and Stabilization —each playing a unique role in sculpting your success. You've delved into the science behind the diet, understanding not only what to eat but why it works. Real-life success stories have served as beacons, illuminating the possibilities and potential that lie ahead.

As you prepare to transition to Book 2, filled with recipes, meal plans, and practical culinary guidance, remember that the Dukan Diet is not just a regimen; it's a lifestyle. It's an invitation to explore the vibrant palette of nutritious foods, engage in culinary creativity, and embrace the joy of well-being.

Your journey is personal, and every step counts. Whether you're embarking on this path for weight loss, health improvement, or a renewed relationship with food, the principles you've learned here will be your steadfast companions. The Dukan Diet is not about deprivation; it's about empowerment, about making choices that align with your goals and nourish your body and soul.

So, as you turn the page to the next chapter of your journey, carry with you the lessons of this book. Let the principles guide you, the phases empower you, and the strategies fortify you. Embrace the promise of a future marked by vitality, balance, and sustained success.

Thank you for entrusting us with a part of your journey. As you continue, may each page turn bring you closer to the transformative and fulfilling life you envision. Here's to your health, your well-being, and the vibrant chapters that lie ahead. Bon voyage!

Do Well to Leave a Review

Dear Dukan Diet Explorer,

Congratulations on completing Book 1 of your Dukan Diet journey! We hope you found inspiration, guidance, and a roadmap to a healthier and more vibrant lifestyle. Your insights are incredibly valuable, not just for us but for others who may be considering embarking on this transformative path.

Why Leave a Review?

1. Inspire Others: Your experience can motivate and inspire others who are contemplating their own wellness journey. Sharing your story could be the nudge someone needs to start their Dukan Diet adventure.

2. Constructive Feedback: Your feedback helps us understand what worked well and where we can improve. Your insights

contribute to refining and enhancing the Dukan Diet experience for future readers.

3. Community Support: By sharing your thoughts, you become part of a supportive community. Your words can encourage fellow Dukan enthusiasts and foster a sense of camaraderie among those on similar paths.

Your contribution matters, and we appreciate the time you take to share your thoughts. Let's build a community that thrives on shared experiences and supports each other in achieving lasting well-being.

Thank you for being an integral part of the Dukan Diet journey!

Below is also my link to join my email list, grab the second bonus and also be among the first to be notified to purchase Book 2

[Link to join the email list]

OR:

https://us21.list-manage.com/contact-form?u=627eb
f11ee9b42d835b71682b&form_id=5e9b51204831f1
8fa6ae6d464061d90e

OR: